GOUT

THE ULTIMATE GOUT COOKBOOK

50 RECIPES FOR INFLAMITORY RELIEF

HR RESEARCH ALLIANCE

Gout Remedies are Through a Proper Diet

My friends, that statement could not be any more true. Many people around the globe today suffer from what is known as gout. Which is a painful form of arthritis that causes inflammation in the joints, mainly in the smaller bones of the feet.

Both men and women can get gout although this does mainly affect men.

Our company HR Research Alliance is here to help if you are a person who may be suffering from this disease.

Like I said, we are here to help. We are not here to make any kind of outlandish claims of curing your gout with our magical elixir or expensive concoction that we came up with in order to market to those who have this painful issue.

This is not what we are about.

We are a team of people who live out in the real world, and we are dedicated to taking real world problems and finding real world solutions for those problems.

We do not over embellish our solutions in order to hoodwink people into purchasing our products. Our only products are books that we sell providing the safest forms of homeopathic remedies that actually can work.

Yes, we not only do extensive research about homeopathic remedies, but we also apply them to our own selves.

Not many companies can say that with a straight face.

If you are reading this now then you already know what gout is and how it can put a damper on your lifestyle.

So we are not going to kill trees and waste your time in the process by creating a page filler Wikipedia style report on the explanation of gout.

You know what gout is already.

If you do not then you will not be looking for gout solutions, hence you would not be reading this right now.

We are trying to help you relieve your gout not teach you an overview of what it is.

So we are going to get to what we do best, and that is providing safe homeopathic remedies that can work if applied properly.

As far as gout is concerned, a persons diet plays a huge role in how extreme the case is or is not of the disease.

Many people will only have minor gout flair ups while others will suffer from gout 24 hours a day.

The later needs to be even more aware of the diet aspect as sometimes just a few small tweaks in the diet can have a major effect on relieving pain.

So we have come up with a cookbook that not only can provide gout relief for some folks, but the recipes are just flat out good for our overall health in general. This cookbook is beneficial to our health on so many levels.

Eating healthy in todays world is not easy for most people. Now add gout flair ups into the mix and you have got yourself an uphill battle to overcome from the starting gates.

We hope that we can do our small part in helping you relieve the pain of gout even if it is only in a minor way.

The main thing when it comes to proper diet is consistency. Sticking with what works is always best for long term results.

We wish you all the best in your quest for gout relief and we thank you for purchasing our gout relief cookbook.

Table of contents

Garlic-Ginger Tofu

Baked Potato with Lentils

Vegan Mac and No-Cheese

Soba Noodles with Spicy Tahini

Spicy Potato Curry

Quinoa Chard Pilaf

Tofu Broccoli Quiche

Lentil and Veggie Bake

Grilled Tomato-Balsamic Veggies with Couscous

Tempeh Fajitas

Lentil, Kale, and Red Onion Pasta

Teriyaki Tofu with Pineapple

Tofu and Red Bell Peppers with Spicy Peanut Sauce

Toasted Almond and Quinoa Salad

Vegan Chili

One-Pot Marrakesh Stew

Crispy Sesame Tofu and Broccoli

Stuffed Sweet Potatoes

Tofu Kebabs with Cilantro Dressing

Four-Grain Vegan Salad

Barley with Winter Greens Pesto

Cajun Style Tempeh Po' Boy

Celery Root Soup

Garbanzo Cakes with Mashed Avocado

Vegan Paella

Spicy Quinoa with Edamame

Avocado Pasta with Blackened Veggies

Black-eyed Peas with Collard Greens and Turnips

Vegan Black Bean Quesadillas

Stuffed Red Bell Pepper

Couscous with Olives and Sun-dried Tomatoes

Braised White Beans and Chard

Miso Soup with Napa Cabbage

Vegan Chinese Porridge

Curried Carrot Soup

Vegan Kofte

Creamy Vegan Alfredo

Note: These recipes are designed to aid in your overall health and wellbeing. These recipes are not written by a Doctor. Always seek your Doctors advice first before adding or taking away anything from your diet. Consult with your Doctor first before applying any of these recipes into your daily life. These recipes are to promote overall health and long lasting wellness. They are not to be mistaken for any type of cure or miracle. We are not promising miracles here nor will we ever do so. We promote a natural approach to overall health. Always check recipes for any types of foods that you may be allergic to prior to eating them.

Tomato Parsley Potatoes

Ingredients:

Potatoes:

- 3-4 red or baby Idaho potatoes, cut into quarters

- ½ Tbsp. extra-virgin olive oil

- ¼ tsp. garlic powder

- ¼ tsp. onion powder

- ¼ tsp. kosher salt

- Pinch of pepper

Tomato-Parsley Reduction Sauce:

- 1 tsp. extra-virgin olive oil

- ½ clove garlic, minced

- 1 Tbsp. diced onion

- 1 can (5.5 oz.) tomato juice

- ½ tsp. cornstarch

- ¾ tsp. horseradish

- ½ Tbsp. ketchup

- ¼ tsp. celery seed

- ¼ tsp. paprika

- ½ Tbsp. lemon juice

- A few dashes of hot sauce, to taste

- Salt & Pepper, to taste

- ¼ cup parsley, chopped

Directions

1. Preheat the oven to 400 degrees F and line a baking sheet with parchment paper.

2. Combine quartered potatoes with the olive oil and spices listed in the first section.

3. Transfer potatoes to prepared baking sheet and spread out evenly. Bake for 35-40 minutes,

flipping the potatoes every 10 minutes or so to ensure even crisping.

4. While the potatoes are roasting, heat olive oil in a saucepan over medium heat. Add garlic and onion; cook, stirring often, for about 3-5 minutes, or until translucent.

5. In a separate bowl, whisk together tomato juice, cornstarch, horseradish, ketchup, celery, seed, paprika, lemon juice and hot sauce until well-combined.

6. Add the tomato mixture to the saucepan with the garlic and onion. Cook 10-15 minutes, stirring occasionally--the mixture will thicken and reduce by almost half. Add salt and pepper to taste.

7. Drizzle the tomato reduction over the roasted potatoes and top with chopped parsley.

Nutritional Information

- Calories: 350

- Total Fat: 4.4g

- Saturated Fat: 0.2g

- Carbohydrates: 73g

- Protein: 4.6g

Creamy Wild Rice Chowder

Ingredients:

- ¼ cup raw cashews, soaked overnight and drained

- ½ medium potato, cooked with skin

- ½ can white beans, rinsed

- 1 tsp. extra-virgin olive oil

- ½ yellow onion, diced

- 2 cloves garlic, minced

- ½ rib celery, diced

- ¼ cup wild rice, not cooked

- ¼ cup brown rice, soaked overnight and drained

- 2 cups vegetable broth (or water)

- ¼ Tbsp. white or yellow miso paste

- 1 Tbsp. white balsamic vinegar (or ½ Tbsp. lemon juice)

- ¼ cup white wine (optional)

- Salt & Pepper, to taste

- ¼ cup fresh parsley, chopped

Directions:

1. Combine cashews, cooked potato, and white beans in a food processor or blender and blend well until completely smooth. If needed, add a little of the water or vegetable broth to blend.

2. Heat oil in a large saucepan or small pot over medium heat. Add the onion, garlic, and celery and a pinch of salt. Stir and continue cooking until soft, about 3-5 minutes.

3. Add the wild rice and brown rice. Stir and cook for another 1-2 minutes

4. Add the vegetable broth and bring the mixture to a boil. Once it boils, reduce the heat to medium.

5. Whisk the miso with a bit of water to thin it out. Add the miso, vinegar, white wine and a pinch of pepper.

6. Stir in the cashew mixture and continue to cook the soup at a steady simmer, stirring frequently to ensure the rice does not stick to the bottom. Add more broth if you would like a thinner chowder.

7. Simmer for 30-45 minutes (until the wild rice is cooked).

8. Season with salt and pepper and top with parsley. Any extra can be stored in an airtight container, in the fridge, for up to a week.

Nutritional Information (for one serving, approximately 1/4th of soup)

- Calories: 175.1

- Total Fat: 4.3g

- Saturated Fat: 0.9g

- Carbohydrates: 28.7g

- Protein: 5.4g

Vegan Bean Burger

Ingredients:

- 1 Tbsp. onion, diced

- 1 Tbsp. grated carrot

- 1 Tbsp. bread crumbs

- 1/4 cup kidney beans, rinsed and drained

- ¼ cup cannellini beans, rinsed and drained

- ½ Tbsp. parsley, finely chopped

- Pinch of chili powder

- Salt and Pepper to taste

- 1 tsp. flour

- 3 Tbsp. Extra Virgin Olive Oil for frying

- Whole wheat hamburger bun

Directions:

1. Put half the breadcrumbs in a mixing bowl.

2. Heat 1 Tbsp. olive oil in a medium saucepan and add onion. Cook for 3 minutes, or until softened and then add the grated carrot and cook for an additional 2-3 minutes. Add onions and carrots the breadcrumbs.

3. In a separate bowl, roughly mash the kidney and cannellini beans with a fork and then stir into the carrot mixture. Add a pinch of chili powder, salt and pepper.

4. In a shallow bowl, combine the remaining breadcrumbs with flour, parsley, salt, and pepper.

5. Shape your bean-carrot blend into 1 or 2 burger patties. Thoroughly coat the patty in the flour mixture.

6. Heat 2 Tbsp. olive oil in a frying pan over medium heat. Carefully add your burger patty

and fry each side until golden brown (about 5 minutes).

7. Place in whole wheat bun, top with desired condiments, and enjoy.

Nutritional Information

- Calories: 225.2

- Total Fat: 1.6g

- Saturated Fat: 0.2g

- Carbohydrates: 44.7g

- Protein: 8g

Swiss Chard with Garbanzo Beans and Couscous

Ingredients:

- 4 Tbsp. couscous

- 2 Tbsp. pine nuts

- 1 Tbsp. Extra Virgin Olive Oil

- 1 clove garlic, thinly sliced

- 5 Tbsp. garbanzo beans, drained and rinsed

- 2 Tbsp. golden raisins (or dark)

- ½ bunch Swiss Chard, stems trimmed

- Salt and Pepper, to taste

Directions:

1. Place the couscous in a large bowl and add 1/3 cup boil water. Stir, cover tightly and let stand for 10 minutes.

2. While the couscous cooks, toast the pine nuts in a large skillet over low heat. Toast for 3-4 minutes, shaking the pan frequently. Set toasted pine nuts aside.

3. Heat olive oil in the skillet over medium heat. Add the garlic and cook until fragrant, about 1 minute.

4. Add the garbanzo beans, raisins, chard, salt and pepper. Cook for about 5 minutes, stirring occasionally, until chard is tender. Remove from heat.

5. Fluff couscous with a fork and place in a bowl or plate. Top with prepared chard, sprinkle with pine nuts, and enjoy.

Nutritional Information

- Calories: 142.4

- Total Fat: 6 g

- Saturated Fat: 0.25 g

- Carbohydrates: 17.8 g

- Protein: 4.3 g

Garbanzo Curry

Ingredients:

- ¾ tsp. extra-virgin olive oil
- ¼ onion, minced
- ½ clove garlic, minced
- ¼ tsp. fresh ginger root, finely chopped
- 1 whole clove
- 1/8 tsp. cinnamon
- 1/8 tsp. ground cumin
- 1/8 tsp ground coriander.
- Pinch of salt
- 1/8 tsp. cayenne pepper
- 1/8 tsp. ground turmeric
- ¼ 15oz-can garbanzo beans, drained and rinsed.

- **2 Tbsp. chopped fresh cilantro**

- **1/4 cup jasmine rice**

- **1/2 cup water**

Directions:

1. First prepare the rice by placing both the rice and water in a medium saucepan or small pot. Turn the heat to high until it begins to boil, and then reduce to low, cover and let simmer for 15 minutes.

2. Heat olive oil in a large frying pan over medium heat for 1 minute. Sauté onions until tender, about 3-4 minutes.

3. Stir in garlic, ginger, clove, cinnamon, cumin, coriander, salt, cayenne, and turmeric. Cook for 1 minute over medium heat, stirring constantly.

4. Add in garbanzo beans and a little bit of water (about ½ Tbsp.).

5. Continue to cook for, stirring occasionally, for about 15-20 minutes, or until all the ingredients are well-blended and cooked through. Remove from heat.

6. Place cooked rice in a bowl, top with garbanzo curry, and garnish with cilantro.

Nutritional Information

- Calories: 294.9

- Total Fat: 4.5g

- Saturated Fat: 0.7g

- Carbohydrates: 56.5g

- Protein: 7.1g

Vegan Polenta Arepas

Ingredients:

- 1/4 (8 oz.) container of tofu, drained

- 1/4 (16oz) tube prepared polenta

- 1/2 Tbsp. Extra virgin olive oil

- 1/2 banana, sliced lengthwise

- 1/4 cup black beans, undrained

- 1/2 avocado, sliced thinly

- 1/4 mango, diced

- 1 Tbsp. diced onion

- 1/4 jalapeno, seeded and diced

- Salt and pepper, to taste

Directions:

1. Preheat the oven's broiler and set the oven rack about 6 inches from the heat source.

2. Slice the tofu and polenta into equal-sized slabs, brush with olive oil and arrange on a greased baking sheet.

3. Cook the tofu and polenta under the broiler until the tops are crispy, about 5 minutes. Remove from onion and set aside.

4. Heat the olive oil in medium skillet over medium-high heat. Sauté the bananas until crispy on the outside, about 5 minutes. Remove from oil and set aside.

5. Place the black beans into a blender and blend until it becomes a thick sauce.

6. In a separate bowl, combine mango, onion, jalapeno, salt and pepper.

7. To arrange, place a slice of polenta on a plate and top with 1/4 of the bean sauce, then tofu, banana, avocado, and then top with the mango salsa and serve.

Nutritional Information

- Calories: 409.9

- Total Fat: 15.5 g

- Saturated Fat: 4.6 g

- Carbohydrates: 54 g

- Protein: 13.6 g

Ginger Stir-Fry with Coconut Rice

Ingredients:

- 1/2 tsp. corn starch

- 1/2 clove garlic, crushed

- 1/2 tsp. chopped fresh ginger root, divided

- 2 tsp. extra virgin olive-oil, divided

- 1/4 cup broccoli florets

- 1 Tbsp. snow peas

- 2 Tbsp. julienned carrots

- 1 Tbsp. red bell pepper, diced

- 1 tsp. soy sauce

- 1 tsp. water

- 1/2 Tbsp. chopped onion

- **1/4 cup jasmine rice**

- **1/4 cup coconut milk**

- **1/4 cup water**

- **Sriracha (or other hot sauce)**

Directions:

1. First prepare the rice by placing the rice, coconut milk, and water in a medium saucepan or small pot. Turn the heat to high until it begins to boil, and then reduce to low, cover and let simmer for 15 minutes, or until most of the coconut milk has been absorbed.

2. In a large bowl, blend cornstarch, garlic, half the ginger, and 1 tsp. olive oil until cornstarch is dissolved.

3. Add the broccoli, snow peas, carrots, and bell pepper, tossing to lighting coat.

4. Heat the remaining olive oil in a wok over medium heat. Add vegetables, cook for 1 minute, stirring constantly to prevent burning.

5. Add onions, salt, remaining ginger, soy sauce and water. Cook until vegetables are tender, but still crisp—about 2 minutes.

6. Place coconut rice in a bowl, top with ginger stir fry. Add Sriracha to taste.

Nutritional Information

- Calories: 338.6

- Total Fat: 16.2 g

- Saturated Fat: 13.1 g

- Carbohydrates: 42 g

- Protein: 6.2 g

Avocado Tacos

Ingredients:

- 1 avocado, peeled, pitted, and mashed

- 2 Tbsp. onions, diced

- 1/8 tsp. garlic salt

- 1 tsp. lemon juice

- Drizzle olive oil

- 2 Tbsp. tomato, diced

- 2 tsp. cilantro, chopped

- Salt and pepper, to taste

- 1/4 cup black beans, drained and rinsed

- 1/2 garlic clove, chopped

- Salt and pepper, to taste

Directions:

1. Preheat oven to 325 degrees F.

2. In a medium saucepan, heat olive oil over medium heat and add the garlic and half the onions and cook until translucent, about 2-5 minutes.

3. Add the black beans, turn heat the low. Stir occasionally and allow the beans to heat while you work on the filling.

4. Arrange corn tortillas in a single layer on a large baking sheet, and place in the preheated oven 2 to 5 minutes, until heated through.

5. In a medium bowl, mix avocado, remaining onion, tomatoes, garlic salt, pepper, lemon juice and a drizzle of olive oil.

6. Spread tortillas with avocado mixture, add black beans and top with cilantro.

Nutritional Information

- Calories: 377.1

- Total Fat: 18.3 g

- Saturated Fat: 3.4g

- Carbohydrates: 43.8 g

- Protein: 9.3 g

Vegan Style Shepherd's Pie

Ingredients:

Mashed potatoes:

- 5 russet potatoes, peeled and cut into 1-inch cubes

- 1/2 cup vegan mayonnaise

- 1/2 cup soy milk (or other milk substitute)

- 1/4 cup olive oil

- 3 Tbsp. vegan cream cheese

- 2 tsp. salt

Filling:

- 2 carrots, diced

- 2 stalks celery, diced

- 3/4 cup broccoli florets

- 1 tsp. Italian seasoning

- 1 clove garlic, minced

- 1/2 tsp. celery seed (optional)

- Pepper, to taste

- 1 (14 oz.) package vegan ground beef substitute

- 1 Tbsp. extra virgin olive oil

- 1 large yellow onion, diced

- 1/2 cup Cheddar-style soy cheese, shredded

Directions:

1. Place potatoes in a large pot, cover with cold water, and bring to a boil over medium-high heat. Turn the heat to medium-low and simmer the potatoes until tender, about 25 minutes. Drain and return to the pot.

2. In a bowl, combine the vegan mayonnaise, soy milk, olive oil, vegan cream cheese, and salt. Add to the potatoes mix with a potato masher until smooth and fluffy. Set aside.

3. Preheat the oven to 400 degrees F and grease a 2-quart baking dish.

4. In a medium skillet, heat the olive oil over medium heat. Add the onions, carrots, celery, and broccoli and cook for 10 minutes, or until softened. Stir in the Italian seasoning, celery seed, garlic, and pepper.

5. Reduce the heat to medium-low and crumble the vegan ground beef substitute into the skillet. Cook and stir, until the mixture is hot, about 5 minutes.

6. Spread the vegetable and "meat" filling into the bottom of the baking dish, and top with the mashed potatoes, smoothing them into an even layer. Top the whole pie with the shredded soy cheese.

7. Bake in a preheated oven until the cheese is melted and slightly browned, approximately 20 minutes. Remove and serve. Leftovers can be stored in an airtight container, in the fridge, for up to a week.

Nutritional Information (for 1/6ᵗʰ of the pie)

- Calories: 558.4

- Total Fat: 24.4 g

- Saturated Fat: 3.6 g

- Carbohydrates: 64.5 g

- Protein: 20.2 g

BBQ Tempeh Sandwiches:

Ingredients:

- 1/4 cup barbeque sauce, any kind

- 1/4 (8 oz.) package tempeh, crumbled

- 3/4 tsp. extra virgin olive oil

- 1/4 red bell pepper, seeded and diced

- 1/4 green bell pepper, seeded and diced

- 1/4 red onion, diced

- 1 Kaiser roll, split and toasted

Directions:

1. Pour the barbeque sauce into a medium bowl and crumble the tempeh into the sauce. Stir until the tempeh is covered, and let marinate for at least 10 minutes.

2. Heat olive oil in a skillet over medium heat. Add the onion, red, and green bell peppers. Cook for 4-5 minutes, stirring frequently.

3. Add the tempeh and barbeque sauce, stir and let cook until tempeh is heated through, about 8-10 minutes.

4. Spoon the bbq tempeh mixture into the toasted Kaiser roll and serve.

Nutritional Information

- Calories: 383.1

- Total Fat: 11.5g

- Saturated Fat: 2.1g

- Carbohydrates: 54.7g

- Protein: 15.2g

Easy Vegan Pasta with Pine Nuts

Ingredients:

- 1/2 cup farfalle pasta

- 1 roma tomato, diced

- 1 Tbsp. extra virgin olive oil

- 1 clove garlic, minced

- 2 Tbsp. fresh basil, cut into thin strips

- Salt and pepper, to taste

- 2 Tbsp. pine nuts

Directions:

1. Bring a small pot of salted water to a boil. Add pasta and cook for 8-10 minutes. Drain.

2. In a large bowl, gently toss the cooked pasta, tomatoes, olive oil, garlic and basil.

3. Season with salt and pepper and top with pine nuts.

Nutritional Information

- Calories: 275.6

- Total Fat: 14.8 g

- Saturated Fat:1.2 g

- Carbohydrates: 32.2 g

- Protein: 3.4 g

Mediterranean Zucchini

Ingredients:

- 1 tsp. extra virgin olive oil

- 2 Tbsp. onion, diced

- 2 Tbsp. red bell pepper, diced

- 1 clove garlic, diced

- 1/4 cup whole peeled tomatoes, chopped

- 1/2 cup finely chopped zucchini

- 1/4 cup cannellini beans, drained

- Pinch oregano

- Salt and pepper, to taste

- 1/4 cup rice, any kind

- 1/2 cup water

Directions:

1. First prepare the rice by placing the rice and water in a medium saucepan or small pot. Turn the heat to high until it begins to boil, and then reduce to low, cover and let simmer for 15 minutes, or until all the water has been absorbed.

2. Heat oil in a small saucepan over medium heat. Stir in onion, red bell pepper, and garlic and cook until fragrant, about 2-5 minutes.

3. Add tomatoes, zucchini, oregano, salt and pepper. Reduce heat, cover, and simmer for 20 minutes, stirring occasionally.

4. Stir in the cannellini beans into the zucchini mixture and continue cooking for 10 minutes.

5. Spoon over the cooked rice and serve.

Nutritional Information

- Calories: 292.3

- Total Fat: 7.5g

- Saturated Fat: 0.9g

- Carbohydrates: 47.2g

- Protein: 9g

Pumpkin-Apple Curry with Lentils

Ingredients:

- 1/3 cup red lentils

- 1/3 cup brown lentils

- 2 1/2 cups water

- 1/8 tsp turmeric

- 1 tsp. extra virgin olive oil

- 1/4 onion, diced

- 3 tomatoes, diced

- 1 clove garlic, minced

- 2 tsp. curry powder

- 3/4 tsp. ground cumin

- 1/8 tsp. salt

- 1/8 tsp. black pepper

- 1/8 tsp. ground cloves

- 2/3 cup peeled and seeded pumpkin, cut into 1-inch cubes

- 1/2 potato, diced

- 1 carrot, diced

- 1 Granny smith apple, cored and diced

Directions:

1. Place the red and brown lentils in a pan with the water and turmeric. Cook over medium-low heat until tender, about 45 minutes. Drain, and reserve 1 cup of the cooking liquid.

2. In a medium pot, heat the oil over medium heat. Stir in the onion, cook until translucent, about 5 minutes. Add in the tomatoes and garlic, cook for 5 minutes, stirring occasionally.

3. Mix in the curry powder, cumin, salt, pepper, and cloves. Add the cooked lentils, reserved cooking liquid, pumpkin, potatoes, and carrots.

Cover and cook over medium-low heat for 35-45 minutes, or until the vegetables are tender.

4. Stir in the apple and lentils. Cook for an additional 15 minutes.

Nutritional Information

- Calories: 199.8

- Total Fat: 3.4 g

- Saturated Fat: 0.1 g

- Carbohydrates: 32.3 g

- Protein: 10.1 g

Garlic-Ginger Tofu

Ingredients:

- 1 tsp. extra virgin olive oil

- 1 garlic clove, minced

- 2 tsp. minced fresh ginger root

- Squeeze of lime juice

- 1/2 tsp. tamari

- 1/4 pound firm tofu

- 1/4 rice, any variety

- 1/2 cup of water

Directions:

1. First prepare the rice by placing the rice and water in a medium saucepan or small pot. Turn the heat to high until it begins to boil, and then reduce to low, cover and let simmer for 15

minutes, or until all the water has been absorbed.

2. Drain tofu with a paper toil and pat dry. Cut into cubes.

3. Heat oil in a wok over medium heat. Stir in garlic and ginger, cook for 1 minute.

4. Add tofu to the pan with tamari, and stir to coat. Cover and continue cooking for 20 minutes.

5. Serve tofu over rice and top with a squeeze of lime juice.

Nutritional Information

- Calories: 243.1

- Total Fat: 3.9g

- Saturated Fat: 1g

- Carbohydrates: 36 g

- Protein: 6g

Baked Potato with Lentils

Ingredients:

- 1 tsp. extra virgin olive oil
- 1/2 white onion, halved and sliced into rings
- 1 garlic clove, minced
- 1/4 cup lentils
- 1 cup water
- 1/2 tsp. salt
- 1/2 tsp. cumin
- Black pepper, to taste
- 1 clove garlic, crushed
- 1 russet potato
- Drizzle of olive oil

Directions:

1. First prepare the baked potato. Preheat the oven to 400 degrees F. Wash the potato and then pierce a few times with a fork, and place it directly on rack in preheated oven and cook for 45 minutes. Place a baking sheet on the rack below to catch any drippings. Once cooked, remove from oven and set aside.

2. Heat olive oil in a heavy pan over medium heat. Sauté the onion for 5 minutes or until it begins to turn golden. Add minced garlic and sauté for another minute.

3. Add lentils and water to the saucepan. Bring the mixture to a boil, then cover, lower the heat, and simmer for 35 minutes, or until the lentils are soft.

4. Add the salt, cumin, and crushed garlic clove to the mixture. Cover and simmer until all is heater and integrated, about 10 minutes.

5. Cut open the baked potato, drizzle with olive oil, and fill with the lentil mixture. Season with salt and pepper and serve.

Nutritional Information

- Calories: 241.5

- Total Fat: 4.3g

- Saturated Fat: 0.2g

- Carbohydrates: 41 g

- Protein: 9.7 g

Vegan Mac and No-Cheese

Ingredients:

- ¾ cup uncooked elbow macaroni
- 1 tsp. extra virgin olive oil
- 2 Tbsp. onion, chopped
- 1 garlic clove, chopped
- ¼ cup cashews
- 1 Tbsp. lemon juice
- 1/3 cup water
- Salt and pepper, to taste
- 1 Tbsp. extra virgin olive oil
- 2 Tbsp. roasted red peppers, drained
- ½ tsp. garlic powder
- ½ tsp. onion powder

Directions:

1. Preheat oven to 350 degrees F.

2. Bring a medium pot of salted water to a boil. Add pasta and cook for 8 to 10 minutes. Drain and transfer to a small baking dish.

3. Heat olive oil in a medium saucepan over medium heat. Stir in onion and garlic and cook until fragrant and lightly browned, about 3-5 minutes. Add to the macaroni.

4. Using a blender or food processor, combine cashews, lemon juice, water and a pinch of salt. Gradually add in 1 Tbsp. olive oil, roasted red peppers, garlic powder and onion powder. Blend until smooth. Mix thoroughly with the macaroni.

5. Bake for 45 minutes in the preheated oven, or until slightly browned on top. Allow to cool 10-15 minutes, top with black pepper and serve.

Nutritional Information

- Calories: 206.6

- Total Fat: 9.8 g

- Saturated Fat: 0.3g

- Carbohydrates: 25.5 g

- Protein: 4.1 g

Soba Noodles with Spicy Tahini

Ingredients:

- ¼ (8 oz.) package dried soba noodles

- 1 tsp. extra virgin olive oil

- 1 clove garlic, minced

- 2 tsp. minced fresh ginger

- ¼ bunch kale, torn into bite-size pieces

Sauce:

- 3 Tbsp. tahini

- 2 tsp. rice vinegar

- 1 ½ tsp. soy sauce

- 1 ½ tsp. extra virgin olive oil

- Drizzle of Sriracha, or other hot sauce

- **Pinch of ground turmeric (or more, to taste)**

- **2 tsp. water**

Directions:

1. To prepare the sauce, use a medium bowl to combine tahini, rice vinegar, soy sauce, 1 ½ tsp. olive oil, Sriracha, turmeric, and 2 tsp. water. Add more water if needed to get the dressing to your preferred consistency; set aside.

2. Bring a pot of lightly salted water to a boil. Cook soba noodles at a boil until tender yet firm to the bite, about 5 to 7 minutes. Drain the noodles; set aside

3. Heat 1 tsp. olive oil in a medium skillet over medium heat. Cook and stir garlic in the olive oil until fragrant, about 1 minute.

4. Add ginger to the garlic and cook 1 minute more.

5. Add kale to the skillet; cook and stir for 1 minute more. Reduce heat to low, cover the skillet, and simmer until the kale wilts, about 5 to 10 minutes.

6. Toss the drained soba noodles in the tahini sauce until coated. Fold the kale into the noodles and sauce and serve.

Nutritional Information

- Calories: 178.7

- Total Fat: 9.9 g

- Saturated Fat: 1.3g

- Carbohydrates: 16.9 g

- Protein: 5.5 g

Spicy Potato Curry

Ingredients:

- 1 large potato, peeled and cubed

- 1 tsp. extra virgin olive oil

- 1 Tbsp. yellow onion, diced

- 1 garlic clove, minced

- ½ tsp. ground cumin

- ½ tsp. cayenne

- ¾ tsp. curry powder

- ¾ tsp. garam masala

- 2 tsp. fresh ginger root, peeled and minced

- Pinch of salt

- 1 tomato, diced

- ¼ cup garbanzo beans, rinsed and drained

- ¼ cup coconut milk

Directions:

1. Place the cubed potato in a small pot and cover with salted water. Bring to a boil over high heat, then reduce heat to medium-low, cover, and simmer until just tender, about 15 minutes. Drain and allow to steam-dry for a minute or two.

2. Heat the olive oil in a medium skillet over medium heat. Add the onion and garlic and cook until the onion has softened and turned translucent, about 5 minutes.

3. Season onion and garlic with with cumin, cayenne pepper, curry powder, garam masala, ginger, and salt; cook for 2 minutes more.

4. Add the tomatoes, garbanzo beans, and potatoes. Pour in the coconut milk, and bring to a simmer. Simmer 5 to 10 minutes. Place in bowl and serve.

Nutritional Information

- Calories: 279.4

- Total Fat: 16.2 g

- Saturated Fat: 13.1 g

- Carbohydrates: 31.4 g

- Protein: 2 g

Quinoa Chard Pilaf

Ingredients:

- 1 tsp. extra virgin olive oil

- 1 Tbsp. onion, diced

- 1 clove garlic, minced

- ¼ cup uncooked quinoa, rinsed

- 2 Tbsp. canned/prepared lentils, rinsed

- ½ cup vegetable broth

- ¼ bunch Swiss chard, stems removed

Directions:

1. Heat the oil in a small pot over medium heat. Stir in the onion and garlic, and sauté until onion is tender, about 5 minutes.

2. Add in quinoa and lentils. Pour in the broth. Cover, and cook 15 minutes.

3. Remove the pot from heat. Shred chard, and gently mix into the pot. Cover, and allow to sit 5 minutes, or until chard is wilted.

4. Serve and enjoy.

Nutritional Information

- Calories: 148.7

- Total Fat: 3.1 g

- Saturated Fat: 0.6 g

- Carbohydrates: 26.6 g

- Protein: 3.6 g

Tofu Broccoli Quiche

Ingredients:

- 1 (9-inch) unbaked vegan pie crust

- 1 large head of broccoli, chopped

- 1 Tbsp. olive oil

- 1 onion, finely chopped

- 4 cloves garlic, minced

- 1 pound firm tofu, drained

- ½ cup soy milk (or preferred milk alternative)

- ¼ tsp. Dijon mustard

- ¾ tsp. salt

- ¼ tsp. ground nutmeg

- ½ tsp. ground red pepper

- **Black pepper to taste**

- **1 Tbsp. dried parsley**

- **1/8 cup parmesan flavor soy cheese**

Directions:

1. Preheat oven to 400 degrees F. Bake pie crust in preheated oven for 10 to 12 minutes.

2. Place broccoli in a steamer over 1 inch of boiling water and cover. Cook until tender but still firm, about 2 to 6 minutes. Drain and set aside.

3. Heat oil in a large skillet over medium-high heat. Sauté onion and garlic until golden, about 3-5 minutes. Stir in the broccoli and cook for an additional minute.

4. In a blender, combine tofu, soy milk, mustard, salt, nutmeg, ground red pepper, black pepper, parsley and Parmesan soy cheese and blend until smooth.

5. In a large bowl combine tofu mixture with broccoli mixture. Pour into pie crust.

6. Bake in preheated oven until quiche is set, about 35 to 40 minutes. Allow to stand for at least 5 minutes before cutting and serving. Leftovers can be stored in an airtight container in the fridge for up to a week.

Nutritional Information (for 1/6th of quiche)

- Calories: 353.6

- Total Fat: 19.6 g

- Saturated Fat: 3.9 g

- Carbohydrates: 26.3 g

- Protein: 18 g

Lentil and Veggie Bake

Ingredients:

- ½ cup long-grain rice, uncooked
- 2 ½ cups water
- 1 cup red lentils
- 1 tsp. olive oil
- 1 small onion, diced
- 3 cloves garlic, minced
- 1 tomato, diced
- 1/3 cup diced celery
- 1/3 cup chopped carrots
- 1/3 cup chopped zucchini
- 1 (8 oz.) can tomato sauce
- 1 tsp. dried basil

- 1 tsp. dried oregano

- 1 tsp. ground cumin

- ½ tsp. celery seed

- **Salt and pepper, to taste**

Directions:

1. Preheat oven to 350 degrees F. In a small bowl, combine basil, oregano, cumin, celery seed, and a pinch of salt and pepper. Set aside.

2. Place the rice and 1 cup water in a medium pot over high heat and bring to a boil. Cover, reduce heat to low, and simmer 20 minutes.

3. Place lentils in a pot with the remaining 1 ½ cups water, and bring to a boil. Cook 15 minutes, or until tender.

4. Heat the oil in a skillet over medium heat, and stir in the onion and garlic. Mix in tomato,

celery, carrots, zucchini, and ½ the tomato sauce. Season with ½ the seasoning mix.

5. In a casserole dish, mix the rice, lentils, and vegetables. Top with remaining tomato sauce, and sprinkle with remaining seasoning.

6. Bake 30 minutes in the preheated oven, until the top is bubbling. Remove and serve. Store leftovers in an airtight container, in the fridge, for up to a week.

Nutritional Information (for 1/6th of bake)

- Calories: 192.7

- Total Fat: 1.5 g

- Saturated Fat: 0.2 g

- Carbohydrates: 35.1 g

- Protein: 9.7 g

Grilled Tomato-Balsamic Veggies with Couscous

Ingredients:

- 1 tsp. olive oil

- ¼ red bell pepper, cut into strips

- ¼ zucchini, cut into thick slices

- ¼ small eggplant, cubed

- ¼ large sweet onion, diced

- 3 Tbsp. frozen broad beans

- 2 tomatoes, diced

- 2 tsp. balsamic vinegar

- ¼ cup couscous

- ¼ cup vegetable stock

Directions:

1. Heat olive oil in a medium grill pan over high heat. When it is very hot, add all the vegetables to the pan. Press down occasionally to get grill lines across them. Turn occasionally to prevent burning. Cook for about 15 minutes, or until the vegetables are evenly browned and cooked through.

2. Add broad beans to the vegetables. Add diced tomatoes and balsamic vinegar. Simmer for a few minutes while you prepare the couscous.

3. Place couscous into a medium bowl. Add boiling vegetable stock, and stir with a fork. Cover and allow 2-3 minutes to become softened. Place couscous in a bowl and top with the vegetables.

Nutritional Information

- Calories: 82.6

- Total Fat: 1.4 g

- Saturated Fat: 0.1 g

- Carbohydrates: 14.8 g

- Protein: 2.7 g

Tempeh Fajitas

Ingredients:

- 1 ½ tsp. olive oil

- ¼ (8 oz.) package tempeh, broken into bite-size pieces

- 2 tsp. soy sauce

- 1 tsp. lime juice

- 1 Tbsp. chopped onion

- 1 clove garlic, minced

- 1/3 cup chopped green bell pepper

- ¾ tsp. chopped green chile peppers

- 1 Tbsp. chopped fresh cilantro

- 2 corn tortillas

Directions:

1. Preheat oven to 350 degrees F.

2. Heat oil in medium skillet over medium heat. Add onion and garlic and cook for 3-5 minutes. Add tempeh with soy sauce and lime juice until tempeh browns.

3. Add bell peppers, chile peppers, and cilantro and turn heat to medium-high and cook for 5-10 minutes, stirring occasionally.

4. Meanwhile, heat the corn tortillas in preheated oven until warm and pliable, about 3-5 minutes.

5. Remove tortillas from oven, fill with tempeh mixture and enjoy.

Nutritional Information

- Calories: 154.7

- Total Fat: 4.3 g

- Saturated Fat: 1.2 g

- Carbohydrates: 23.2 g

- Protein: 5.8 g

Lentil, Kale, and Red Onion Pasta

Ingredients:

- ½ cup vegetable broth

- 2 Tbsp. dry lentils

- Pinch of salt

- ½ bay leaf

- 1 Tbsp. olive oil

- ¼ large red onion, chopped

- ¼ tsp. chopped fresh time

- ¼ tsp. dried oregano

- Salt and pepper, to taste

- 1 piece vegan sausage, cut into ¼ inch slices (optional)

- ¼ bunch kale, stems removed and leaves coarsely chopped

- **1 cup rotini pasta**

Directions:

1. Bring the vegetable broth, lentils, pinch of salt, and bay leaf to a boil in a saucepan over high heat. Reduce heat to medium-low, cover, and cook until the lentils are tender, about 20 minutes. Add additional broth if needed to keep the lentils moist. Discard the bay leaf once done.

2. As the lentils simmer, heat the olive oil in a skillet over medium-high heat. Stir in the onion, thyme, oregano, salt, and pepper. Cook and stir for 1 minute, then add the sausage. Reduce the heat to medium-low, and cook until the onion has softened, about 10 minutes.

3. Meanwhile, bring a large pot of lightly salted water to a boil over high heat. Add the kale and rotini pasta. Cook until the rotini is al dente,

about 8 minutes. Remove some of the cooking water, and set aside. Drain the pasta, then return to the pot,

4. Stir in the lentils and onion mixture. Use the reserved cooking liquid to adjust the moistness of the dish to your liking and serve.

Nutritional Information

- Calories: 184.5

- Total Fat: 4.1 g

- Saturated Fat: 0.5 g

- Carbohydrates: 27.9 g

- Protein: 9 g

Teriyaki Tofu with Pineapple

Ingredients:

- ¼ (12 oz.) package firm tofu

- 1/3 cup chopped fresh pineapple

- ½ cup teriyaki sauce

- ¼ cup rice (any variety)

- ½ cup water

Directions:

1. Cut the tofu into bite-size pieces and place in a baking dish. Add pineapple and pour in teriyaki sauce. Cover and refrigerate for at least 1 hour

2. Preheat oven to 350 degrees F.

3. Bake tofu in preheated oven for 20 minutes, or until hot and bubbly.

4. While the tofu is baking, prepare the rice by placing both the rice and water in a medium saucepan or small pot. Turn the heat to high until it begins to boil, and then reduce to low, cover and let simmer for 15 minutes.

5. Place rice in a bowl and top with pineapple teriyaki tofu.

Nutritional Information

- Calories: 211.5

- Total Fat: 1.9 g

- Saturated Fat: 0 g

- Carbohydrates: 43.1 g

- Protein: 5.5 g

Tofu and Red Bell Peppers with Spicy Peanut Sauce

Ingredients:

- 1/2 package (14 oz.) firm or extra-firm tofu

- 1/2 Tbsp. olive oil

- 1/2 Tbsp. soy sauce, divided

- 1/2 medium red bell pepper, seeded, cut into strips

- 1 Tbsp. onion, diced

- 3/4 Tbsp. smooth peanut butter

- 1/2 Tbsp. fresh lime juice

- 2 tsp. Sriracha or other chili-garlic sauce

- 2 tsp. brown sugar

- 3/4 Tbsp. water

- 1/2 Tbsp. cilantro, chopped (optional)

Directions:

1. Preheat oven to 450 degrees F. Slice tofu into 4 rectangles.

2. In a shallow bowl, whisk together half the olive oil and half the soy sauce. Dip tofu pieces on all sides to coat.

3. Brush a baking sheet with a little bit of olive and place tofu pieces on the baking sheet. Scatter peppers and onions around the edges.

4. Bake 10 minutes; turn tofu, peppers and onions over and continue baking until tofu is golden brown and the vegetables begin to car, about 10-15 minutes more.

5. In a small saucepan over low heat, whisk together peanut butter, lime juice, chili sauce, brown sugar, water, and remaining soy sauce, until warm.

6. Remove tofu, peppers, and onion from oven and place in a bowl or on a plate. Drizzle peanut sauce over them and garnish with cilantro.

Nutritional Information

- Calories: 275

- Total Fat: 11 g

- Saturated Fat: 1 g

- Carbohydrates: 26.4 g

- Protein: 17.6 g

Toasted Almond and Quinoa Salad

Ingredients:

- **3 Tbsp. slivered almonds**

- **1/4 cup quinoa**

- **1/2 cup water**

- **2 tsp. olive oil**

- 1/2 yellow bell pepper, seeded and cut into 1/2 inch chunks

- 1 garlic clove, minced

- 1 scallion, thinly sliced

- Pinch of red pepper flakes

- 1 tsp. chopped fresh thyme

- 1/2 medium zucchini, cut lengthwise and sliced into 1/2 –inch thick pieces

- 1/2 large celery stalk, diced

- Juice from half a lime

- Salt and pepper, to taste

Directions:

1. Preheat oven to 350 degrees. Place almonds on a baking sheet and toast in the oven until crisp, lightly browned, and fragrant, about 7 minutes. Remove from oven and set aside.

2. In a medium saucepan, heat 1 tsp. olive oil over medium heat. Add yellow pepper, garlic, scallions, and red-pepper flakes; cook until the pepper is tender, about 5 minutes.

3. Stir in quinoa, thyme, water, and a pinch of salt. Bring to a boil, reduce to a simmer, cover, and cook 7 minutes.

4. Stir in zucchini, cover, and cook until quinoa is tender but not mushy, 5 to 8 minutes longer. Remove the saucepan from heat.

5. Stir in celery, almonds, and remaining tsp. of olive oil. Season with salt and pepper, fluff with a fork. Serve warm or cold and season with a squeeze of lime right before serving.

Nutritional Information

- Calories: 277.5

- Total Fat: 7.9 g

- Saturated Fat: 1 g

- Carbohydrates: 43.6 g

- Protein: 8 g

Vegan Chili

Ingredients:

- 2 Tbsp. extra virgin olive oil

- 1 medium yellow onion, diced

- 4 garlic cloves, minced

- 1 1/2 tsp. ground cumin

- 1 tsp. chili powder

- Salt and pepper, to taste

- 1 medium zucchini, diced into 1/2-inch cubes

- 3/4 cup tomato paste

- 1 can (15 oz.) black beans, rinsed and drained

- 1 can (15 oz.) pinto beans, rinsed and drained

- 1 can (14 oz.) diced tomatoes with green chiles

- 1 can (14.5 oz.) diced tomatoes

- 2 cups water

Directions:

1. In a large pot, heat oil over medium-high. Add onion and garlic; cook, stirring frequently, until fragrant, about 4 minutes. Add cumin and chili powder, a pinch of salt and pepper, and cook, 1 minute.

2. Add zucchini and tomato paste; cook, stirring frequently, 3 minutes.

3. Add in black beans, pinto beans, and both cans diced tomatoes. Add 2 cups water and bring mixture to a boil. Reduce heat to medium, simmer and cook until zucchini is tender and liquid reduces slightly, about 20 minutes. Season with salt and pepper and serve. Extras

can be stored in an airtight container, in the fridge, for up to a week.

Nutritional Information (per serving, approximately 1/4th of chili)

- Calories: 235.5

- Total Fat: 3.9 g

- Saturated Fat: 0.7 g

- Carbohydrates: 41.1 g

- Protein: 9 g

One-Pot Marrakesh Stew

Ingredients:

- 1 Tbsp. extra-virgin olive oil

- 1 large red onion, diced

- 2 tsp ground cumin

- 1 tsp ground cinnamon

- 1 tsp ground coriander

- 3/4 tsp cayenne pepper

- 1/2 tsp ground allspice

- 4 large carrots, cut into 1-inch pieces

- 2 russet potatoes, peeled and cut into 1-inch pieces

- 1 small butternut squash, peeled, seeded, and cut into 1-inch pieces

- Salt and pepper, to taste

- 1 can (14.5 ounces) diced tomatoes

- 3 3/4 cups vegetable broth

- 2 small eggplants, cut into 1-inch pieces

- 1 can (15.5 ounces) garbanzo beans, rinsed and drained

- 4 Tbsp. couscous

- 1/3 cup boiled water

Directions:

1. Place the couscous in a large bowl and add 1/3 cup boiled water. Stir, cover tightly and let stand for 10 minutes.

2. In an 8-quart Dutch oven or heavy pot, heat oil over medium-high. Add onion and cook, stirring occasionally, until soft, 5 minutes.

3. Add cumin, cinnamon, coriander, cayenne, and allspice and cook until fragrant, 1 minute.

4. Add carrots, potatoes, and squash and season with salt and pepper. Cook, stirring occasionally, until beginning to brown, 5 minutes. Add tomatoes and broth—be sure vegetables are completely covered. If not, add water. Bring to a gentle simmer and cook, uncovered, 20 minutes.

5. Add eggplant, stir to combine, and simmer until eggplant is tender, about 20 minutes more. Stir in chickpeas, season to taste with salt and pepper, and cook until garbanzo beans are warmed through, 3 to 5 minutes.

6. Serve stew with couscous. Leftovers can be stored in an airtight container, in the fridge for up to a week, or frozen, for up to a month.

Nutritional Information (for one serving, approx. 1/6th of stew, with couscous)

- Calories: 234.3

- Total Fat: 5.9 g

- Saturated Fat: 0.3 g

- Carbohydrates: 41 g

- Protein: 4.3 g

Crispy Sesame Tofu and Broccoli

Ingredients:

- 1/2 block firm tofu

- 1 Tbsp. sesame seeds

- 1/4 Tbsp. sesame oil

- 3/4 Tbsp. soy sauce

- 1 cup broccoli, cut into 1/2 inch pieces

- 2 Tbsp. water

- Salt and pepper, to taste

Directions:

1. Slice tofu lengthwise into 2 equal pieces, then down the middle to make 4 squares. Pat squares dry with a paper towel, pressing to help remove more liquid if needed.

2. Spread the sesame seeds on a plate. Press both sides of each tofu square into sesame seeds. In a large nonstick skillet, heat sesame oil over medium heat. Cook tofu, until golden brown, 4 to 6 minutes per side.

3. Add the soy sauce and continue cooking and turning the tofu, until it has absorbed all the liquid, about 1 minute. Remove from pan and set aside.

4. Add broccoli, 2 Tbsp. water, and a pinch of salt and pepper to skillet. Simmer, covered, until broccoli is tender, about 5 minutes.

5. Place broccoli and tofu on a plate, drizzle with additional sesame oil, if desired and serve.

Nutritional Information

- Calories: 148

- Total Fat: 5 g

- Saturated Fat: 1.8 g

- Carbohydrates: 18 g

- Protein: 14 g

Stuffed Sweet Potatoes

Ingredients:

- 1 large round sweet potato

- 1/4 Tbsp. olive oil

- 1/4 small onion, chopped

- 1 garlic clove, minced

- 1/2 tsp. finely chopped rosemary

- Pinch of crushed red pepper flakes

- Salt and pepper, to taste

- 1 cup kale, trimmed and thinly sliced

- 1/8 (14 oz. package) firm tofu, cut into 1/2 –inch cubes

- 2 Tbsp. water

Directions:

1. Preheat oven to 375 degrees F. Line a rimmed baking sheet with parchment paper. Bake sweet potato on sheet until tender but not completely cooked through, 55 minutes to 1 hour. Leave oven on.

2. Once the potato is cool enough to handle, cut off the top quarter and discard. Scoop out and reserve flesh, leaving a 1/2-inch-thick shell; set shells aside. Coarsely chop the flesh; set aside.

3. Heat oil in a large nonstick skillet over medium-high heat. Add onion, garlic, rosemary, salt, and red pepper flakes; cook, stirring occasionally, about 3 minutes. Add kale; cook, stirring occasionally, until kale has wilted, about 5 minutes. Stir in reserved chopped sweet potatoes, the tofu, and water. Cook for an additional minute.

4. Place sweet potato shell on a baking sheet. Spoon filling into shell and cover with foil. Bake until heated through, about 30 minutes. Serve

Nutritional Information

- Calories: 190.5

- Total Fat: 4.5 g

- Saturated Fat: 0.6 g

- Carbohydrates: 32 g

- Protein: 5.5 g

Tofu Kebabs with Cilantro Dressing

Ingredients:

- 1/2 cup fresh cilantro

- 1 Tbsp. olive oil

- 1/4 small jalapeno, seeded

- 1 tsp. grated fresh ginger

- 1/2 Tbsp. fresh lime juice

- 1 scallion, white and green parts separated and cut into 1-inch lengths

- Salt and pepper, to taste

- 1/2 package (14 oz.) extra-firm tofu, cut into 3-4 pieces

- 1/2 summer squash, cut into 1-inch pieces

Directions:

1. Heat grill to medium. In a food processor, combine cilantro, oil, jalapeno, ginger, lime juice, and scallion greens. Blend until smooth; season with salt and pepper.

2. In a bowl, combine tofu, scallion whites, and a drizzle of olive oil; season with salt and pepper. Thread tofu and scallion whites onto 1 skewer, and then thread squash onto 1 skewer.

3. Clean and lightly oil hot grates. Grill squash kebab, covered, until tender, 11 to 13 minutes, turning occasionally. Grill tofu kebab until scallions are soft, about 4 to 6 minutes, turning occasionally.

4. Brush both with cilantro sauce and grill 30 seconds more. Serve kebabs with remaining cilantro sauce.

Nutritional Information

- Calories: 254

- Total Fat: 10 g

- Saturated Fat: 1 g

- Carbohydrates: 27 g

- Protein:14 g

Four-Grain Vegan Salad

Ingredients:

- ¼ cup amaranth seeds
- ¼ cup vegetable broth
- ¼ cup quinoa
- ½ cup vegetable broth
- ¼ cup millet
- ½ cup vegetable broth
- ¼ cup cooked brown basmati or jasmine rice
- ¼ tsp. grated orange zest
- ¼ cup fresh orange segments
- ¼ cup diced fennel
- ¼ cup diced radishes
- 1 Tbsp. olive oil

- **2 Tbsp. fresh orange juice**

- **½Tbsp. red wine vinegar**

- **¼ Tbsp. chopped fresh fennel fronds**

- **Pinch fresh dill**

- **Salt and Pepper, to taste**

Directions:

1. To cook the amaranth—place a small saucepan over medium high heat, add the amaranth. Toast for 4-5 minutes. While amaranth is cooking, bring ¼ cup broth to boil in a medium saucepan. Add amaranth and a pinch of salt to the broth and cover; reduce the heat to simmer for 7 minutes. Remove from heat and set aside.

2. To cook the quinoa—Bring ½ cup vegetable broth and pinch of salt and pepper to a boil in a medium saucepan. Add the quinoa, cover the pan and reduce the heat. Simmer until liquid

has been absorbed, about 7-12 minutes. Set aside.

3. To cook the millet-- place a small saucepan over medium high heat, add the millet. Toast for 4-5 minutes. Remove pan from heat, pour millet into a bowl and add cold water. Swirl and drain. Bring ¼ cup broth to boil in a medium saucepan. Add millet and a pinch of salt to the broth and cover; reduce the heat to simmer for 15 minutes. Remove from heat and set aside.

4. Combine all the prepared ingredients in a large bowl. Refrigerate, covered, for at least 1 hour or as long as 3 to 4 days before serving.

5. Remove from the refrigerator and serve at room temperature.

Nutritional Information

- Calories: 379

- Total Fat: 7 g

- Saturated Fat: 1.9 g

- Carbohydrates: 68 g

- Protein:11 g

Barley with Winter Greens Pesto

Ingredients:

- ½ cup hulled barley

- ¾ cup water

- ½ bunch Swiss Chard, stems removed

- ½ bunch mustard greens, stems removed

- 2 Tbsp. almonds, toasted

- 1 ½ tsp. sherry vinegar

- 1 garlic clove, minced

- 1 ½ Tbsp. walnut oil

- Salt and pepper

Directions:

1. Place the barley, a pinch of salt, and water in a medium saucepan. Bring to a boil over high

heat, and then reduce the heat to low and simmer, covered, until the barley is tender but still slightly chewy, about 30 to 45 minutes. Drain and set aside to cool.

2. Bring a medium saucepan of salted water to a boil over high heat. Add the chard and mustard greens and blanch for 1 minute or until wilted and tender. Drain and let cool slightly.

3. Place the cooled greens, almonds, vinegar, and garlic in a food processor. Add the walnut oil in a steady stream until all of the ingredients are evenly incorporated, about 2 minutes. Scrape down the sides of the bowl, season with salt and pepper, and process until smooth.

4. Place the reserved barley in a large bowl, add the pesto, and mix to combine. Season with salt and pepper and serve.

Nutritional Information

- Calories: 314

- Total Fat: 14 g

- Saturated Fat: 1 g

- Carbohydrates: 37 g

- Protein:10 g

Cajun Style Tempeh Po' Boy

Ingredients:

- ½ (8 oz.) package tempeh, sliced horizontally into ½-inch pieces

- 2 Tbsp. olive oil

- ¼ large yellow onion, thinly sliced

- ½ tsp. garlic powder

- ½ tsp. paprika

- ½ tsp. chili powder

- Pinch red chili flakes

- Pinch cayenne pepper

- ½ tsp. dried thyme

- ½ tsp. dried oregano

- Salt and pepper

- ½ large green bell pepper, seeds removed, cut into long ¼-inch wide strips

- ½ cup water

- 2 Tbsp. tomato paste

- Drizzle pure maple syrup

- Drizzle balsamic vinegar

- 2 tomatoes, diced

- Whole wheat bread roll (or preferred bread)

Directions:

1. Preheat oven to 350°F.

2. In a medium bowl combine the tempeh pieces with a 1/2 Tbsp. of the olive oil and toss well.

3. Heat 1 ½ Tbsp. of the olive oil in a medium skillet over medium-high heat. Add the tempeh fingers and cook for 5 to 7 minutes, adding

more oil if necessary, until lightly browned. Turn the fingers over and cook for 5 to 7 minutes more, until lightly browned on the other side. Transfer the tempeh to a large plate lined with paper towels.

4. Combine ½ Tbsp. of the olive oil with the onion, garlic powder, paprika, chili powder, red chili flakes, cayenne, thyme, oregano, pinch of salt and pepper in a large nonstick skillet over medium-low heat. Slowly sauté for 15 minutes, stirring often to prevent burning, until well caramelized.

5. Add the green bell peppers to the skillet, and sauté for 10 more minutes, or until the bell peppers are softened.

6. In a large bowl combine ½ cup water, tomato paste, maple syrup, vinegar, and a pinch of salt. Whisk well. Add the diced tomatoes with their juices and onion and green pepper mixture. Stir well.

7. Place the tempeh in a small casserole dish. Pour the sauce on top, covering all the tempeh fingers.

8. Cover the dish with foil and bake for 45 minutes, or until most of the sauce is absorbed.

9. Cut bread roll open, if needed. Place tempeh pieces on one slice, making sure you cover it with plenty of sauce, and place another slice on top

Nutritional Information

- Calories: 356

- Total Fat: 12 g

- Saturated Fat: 1 g

- Carbohydrates: 42 g

- Protein: 20g

Celery Root Soup

Ingredients:

- 3 Tbsp. extra-virgin olive oil

- 1 cup thinly sliced, white and light green parts only

- 3 medium celery root, (also known as celeriac), peeled and cut into 1-inch chunks

- 2 large Yukon Gold potatoes, peeled and cut into 1-inch chunks

- 1 Granny Smith apple (or other tart variety), peeled, cored, and cut into 1-inch chunks

- 2 garlic cloves, peeled and smashed

- 2 tsp. salt, plus more as needed

- black pepper

- **3 cups water**

- **2 cups vegetable broth**

Directions:

1. Heat oil in a large saucepan with a tightfitting lid over medium-high heat until shimmering.

2. Add leek and cook, stirring occasionally, until softened and translucent, about 3 minutes. Add celery root, potatoes, apple, garlic, salt, and a pinch of pepper. Stir to coat vegetables with oil.

3. Add water and broth, and bring to a boil. Cover, reduce heat to low, and simmer until vegetables just give way when pierced with a knife, about 20 to 25 minutes.

4. Remove 1 cup of liquid from the saucepan; set aside. Using a blender, purée the soup in batches until smooth, removing the small cap from the blender lid and covering the space with a kitchen towel (this allows steam from the

hot soup to escape and prevents the blender lid from popping off).

5. Once blended, transfer the soup back to the saucepan and keep warm over low heat. If the soup is too thick, add the reserved liquid a little at a time until the soup reaches the desired consistency.

6. Taste and season with additional salt and pepper as needed and serve. Leftover soup can be stored in an airtight container, in the fridge, for up to a week.

Nutritional Information (per serving, 1/4th of soup)

- Calories: 151

- Total Fat: 4.2 g

- Saturated Fat: 0.1 g

- Carbohydrates: 27 g

- Protein:1.3 g

Garbanzo Cakes with Mashed Avocado

Ingredients:

- ¼ cup bulgur wheat

- 1 cup water

- ¼ cup loosely packed parsley leaves

- ¼ cup loosely packed mint leaves

- ¼ cup loosely packed cilantro leaves

- 1 medium clove garlic, roughly chopped

- ¼ teaspoon ground coriander

- ½ serrano or jalapeño chili, stemmed, seeded, and roughly chopped

- ½ can (15 ounce) can of garbanzo beans, drained and rinsed

- Salt and Pepper

- ¼ cup flour

- ¼ cup water

- ¾ vegan panko-style breadcrumbs

- ¼ cup olive oil

- ½ avocado

- ½ Tbsp. lime juice

Directions:

1. Bring 1 cup of water to a boil over high heat. Add bulgur wheat and cook until tender, about 10 minutes. Drain carefully.

2. While wheat cooks, combine parsley, mint, cilantro, garlic, jalapeño and coriander in a food processor. Pulse until finely chopped, scraping down sides as necessary, about 10 to 12 short pulses. Add half garbanzo beans and pulse until a rough puree is formed, scraping down sides as necessary, about 8 to 10 short pulses. Transfer to a bowl.

3. Add remaining chickpeas to food processor and pulse until roughly chopped, 4 to 6 pulses. Transfer to bowl with chickpea/herb mixture. When bulgur wheat has drained, add to bowl. Season with salt and pepper, then fold mixture together, starting with a rubber spatula, and finishing by hand when cool enough to handle. Form mixture into patties roughly 3/4-inch thick and 3 inches wide (you should be able to make 2-3 patties)

4. Combine flour and water in a mcdium bowl and whisk until smooth. Place breadcrumbs in a second bowl.

5. Working one patty at a time, dip in flour mixture to coat, then transfer to breadcrumbs. Cover with breadcrumbs on all sides, and transfer to a plate. Repeat with remaining patties.

6. Put half of oil in a large cast iron or non-stick skillet over medium-high heat until

shimmering. Add the patties in a single layer and cook, swirling pan occasionally, until golden brown on bottoms, about 2 minutes. Carefully flip and cook second side, swirling pan occasionally as they cook, about 2 minutes longer.

7. Place avocado in a small bowl and mash the flesh with a fork. Season with salt and add lime juice. Serve fried chickpea patties with mashed avocado, sliced onions, herbs, and lime or lemon wedges.

Nutritional Information

- Calories: 696.8

- Total Fat: 28 g

- Saturated Fat: 4 g

- Carbohydrates: 96 .2 g

- Protein: 15 g

Vegan Paella

Ingredients:

- 1/2 cup boiling water
- ¼ cup white rice
- ¾ tsp. olive oil
- ¼ onion, chopped
- 1 garlic clove, minced
- ¼ green bell pepper, sliced
- ¼ red bell pepper, sliced
- ½ tomato, diced
- ½ cup vegetable broth
- 1 tsp. paprika
- ½ tsp. ground turmeric
- ¼ cup peas

- ¼ **cup drained and quartered canned artichoke hearts**

- **Salt and pepper**

Directions:

1. Mix boiling water and rice together in a bowl; let stand for 20 minutes. Drain.

2. Heat olive oil in a large skillet over medium heat; cook and stir onion and garlic until onion is transparent, about 5 minutes. Add green bell pepper, red bell pepper, and tomato; cook and stir until peppers are slightly tender, about 3 minutes.

3. Mix rice and vegetable broth into onion-pepper mixture; bring to a boil. Reduce heat to low and simmer. Add paprika, turmeric and a pinch of salt and pepper; cover skillet and simmer until rice is tender, about 20 minutes.

4. Stir peas and artichoke hearts into rice mixture and cook until heated through, about 1 minute more. Serve hot.

Nutritional Information

- Calories: 124.8

- Total Fat: 1.6g

- Saturated Fat: 0.2 g

- Carbohydrates: 25.5 g

- Protein: 2.1g

Spicy Quinoa with Edamame

Ingredients:

- ¾ cup water

- ½ cup quinoa

- 1 tsp. vegetable bouillon

- ¾ cup shelled edamame

- 1 tsp. olive oil

- ½ sweet onion, diced

- ½ bell pepper, diced

- 1 ½ tsp. minced fresh ginger

- 2 garlic cloves, minced

- 1 Tbsp. soy sauce

- 2 tsp. chopped fresh cilantro

- 1 tsp. Sriracha, or other hot chili paste

Directions:

1. Bring water, quinoa, and vegetable bouillon to a boil in a medium pot; stir in edamame, cover, and simmer until quinoa is tender, 15 to 20 minutes.

2. Heat olive oil in a medium skillet over medium heat; cook and stir onions and bell peppers until onions are translucent, about 5 minutes.

3. Add ginger and garlic; cook and stir until fragrant, about 2 minutes. Remove from heat; stir in soy sauce, cilantro, and chili paste.

4. Combine onion mixture and quinoa mixture; simmer, stirring occasionally, until excess broth has been absorbed, about 5 minutes. Serve.

Nutritional Information

- Calories: 165.8

- Total Fat: 5 g

- Saturated Fat: 0.6 g

- Carbohydrates: 21.4 g

- Protein: 8.8 g

Avocado Pasta with Blackened Veggies

Ingredients:

Veggies:

- ¼ head broccoli, cut into 1-inch florets

- ½ red bell pepper, cut into ½ inch chunks

- ¼ yellow onion, thinly sliced into rings

- 2 tsp. olive oil

- Juice from half a lime

- Pinch of salt

Sauce:

- 1 avocado, peeled and chopped

- Juice from ½ lime

- 1 garlic clove, peeled

- 2 Tbsp. chopped fresh cilantro

- **Salt and pepper**

Pasta:

- **1 ½ cup penne pasta**

- **Pinch of salt**

Directions:

1. Preheat oven to 450 degrees F.

2. Combine broccoli, red bell peppers, and yellow onion in a large bowl. Add olive oil, juice from ½ a lime, and a pinch of salt; toss to coat. Spread vegetables onto a baking sheet.

3. Roast vegetables for 30 minutes, stirring 1 or 2 times, until edges begin to blacken. Remove from oven and cool slightly.

4. Fill a large pot with water and a pinch of salt; bring to a boil. Stir in penne and return to a boil. Cook pasta uncovered, stirring

occasionally, until cooked through but still firm to the bite, about 11 minutes; drain.

5. Blend avocado, juice from ½ a lime, garlic, and pinch of salt and pepper in a food processor or blender until sauce is smooth, scraping down sides as needed. Add chopped cilantro and pulse until just incorporated.

6. Gently toss pasta, roasted vegetables, and sauce together in a bowl. Serve.

Nutritional Information

- Calories: 326.7

- Total Fat: 11.5 g

- Saturated Fat: 1.2 g

- Carbohydrates: 45.6 g

- Protein: 10.2 g

Black-eyed Peas with Collard Greens and Turnips

Ingredients:

- ¼ cup brown rice

- ½ cup water

- ½ cup dried black-eye peas

- 1 cup water, or as needed to cover peas

- 1 tsp. soy margarine

- ½ turnip, peeled and chopped

- ¼ bunch collard greens, chopped

- Salt and pepper

- 1 garlic clove, minced

- 1 tomato, chopped

- 1 tsp. balsamic vinaigrette salad dressing

- 1 tsp olive oil (optional)

Directions:

1. Place black-eyed peas into a medium container and cover with several inches of cool water; let stand 8 hours to overnight. Drain and rinse.

2. Prepare the rice by placing both the rice and ½ cup water in a medium saucepan or small pot. Turn the heat to high until it begins to boil, and then reduce to low, cover and let simmer for 15 minutes.

3. In a small pot, cover black-eyed peas with fresh water. Bring to a boil over high heat, then reduce the heat to medium-low; cover and simmer until peas are tender, 40 to 60 minutes. Drain.

4. Heat soy margarine in a skillet over medium heat. Add turnip and collard greens a pinch of salt and pepper; cook for 2 minutes.

5. Stir black-eyed peas, garlic, and tomatoes into collard mixture; cook and stir until collards are tender, about 5 minutes.

6. Season with balsamic vinaigrette and olive oil and serve.

Nutritional Information

- Calories: 159

- Total Fat: 2.6 g

- Saturated Fat: 0.3 g

- Carbohydrates: 30.9 g

- Protein: 3 g

Vegan Black Bean Quesadillas

Ingredients:

- ¼ (15 oz.) can great Northern beans, drained and rinsed
- 4 Tbsp. diced tomatoes
- 1 clove garlic, minced
- ½ tsp. ground cumin
- Pinch of chili powder
- Pinch cayenne pepper
- ¼ cup black beans, drained and rinsed
- Pinch of salt
- 2 whole grain tortillas
- 1 Tbsp. fresh, chopped cilantro
- 1 tsp. olive oil

Directions:

1. Blend great Northern beans, 3 Tbsp. tomatoes, and garlic in a food processor until smooth; add cumin, chili powder, pinch of salt and cayenne and blend again.

2. Transfer bean mixture to a bowl. Stir black beans, 1 Tbsp. tomatoes, and cilantro into bean mixture.

3. Heat oil in skillet over medium-high heat. Place a tortilla in the hot oil. Spread about bean filling onto the tortilla.

4. Place another tortilla on top of filling; cook until filling is warmed, about 10 minutes.

5. Flip quesadilla to cook the second side until lightly browned, 3 to 5 minutes.

Nutritional Information

- Calories: 121.9

- Total Fat: 1.5 g

- Saturated Fat: 0.3 g

- Carbohydrates: 21.4 g

- Protein: 5.7 g

Stuffed Red Bell Pepper

Ingredients:

- ¼ cup brown rice

- ½ cup water

- 1 red bell pepper, top and seeds removed

- 1 tsp olive oil

- ¼ onion, chopped

- 1 garlic clove, chopped

- ¼ (15 oz.) can black-eyed peas, rinsed and drained

- 1 large Swiss Chard leaf, chopped

- Salt and pepper, to taste

Directions:

1. Preheat oven to 350 degrees F. Spray a baking sheet with cooking spray.

2. Bring the brown rice and water to a boil in a saucepan over high heat. Reduce the heat to medium-low, cover, and simmer until the rice is tender and the liquid has been absorbed, 15-30 minutes.

3. Place the red pepper on the prepared baking sheet, and bake until tender, about 15 minutes.

4. Heat the olive oil in a skillet over medium heat, cook and stir the onion and garlic until the onion is translucent, about 5 minutes.

5. Stir in the black-eyed peas and chard. Bring the mixture to a simmer, and cook until the chard is wilted, 5 to 8 minutes. Mix in the cooked brown rice, sprinkle with salt and pepper to taste, and lightly stuff the mixture into the red pepper. Serve hot.

Nutritional Information

- Calories: 100

- Total Fat: 0.8 g

- Saturated Fat: 0.1 g

- Carbohydrates: 20.8 g

- Protein: 2.4 g

Couscous with Olives and Sun-dried Tomatoes

Ingredients:

- ½ cup vegetable broth, divided

- ¼ cup water

- ½ cup pearl couscous

- Pinch salt and pepper

- 1 Tbsp. and 1 tsp olive oil, divided

- 2 Tbsp. pine nuts

- 1 clove garlic, minced

- ¼ shallot, minced

- 2 Tbsp. sliced black olives

- 1 Tbsp. sun- dried tomatoes packed in oil, drained and chopped

- 1 Tbsp. chopped fresh parsley

Directions:

1. Bring ¼ cup vegetable broth and water to a boil in a saucepan, stir in couscous, and mix in salt and black pepper. Reduce heat to low and simmer until liquid is absorbed, about 8 minutes.

2. Heat 1 tsp. olive oil in a skillet over medium-high heat; stir in pine nuts and cook, stirring frequently, until pine nuts smell toasted and are golden brown, about 1 minute. Remove from heat.

3. Heat remaining 1 Tbsp. olive oil in a saucepan; cook and stir garlic and shallot in the hot oil until softened, about 2 minutes. Stir black olives and sun-dried tomatoes into garlic mixture and cook until heated through, 2 to 3 minutes, stirring often.

4. Slowly pour in remaining vegetable broth and bring mixture to a boil. Reduce heat to low and

simmer until sauce has reduced, 8 to 10 minutes.

5. Transfer couscous to a bowl, mix with sauce, and serve topped with parsley and pine nuts.

Nutritional Information

- Calories: 142.1

- Total Fat: 7.3 g

- Saturated Fat: 1 g

- Carbohydrates: 15.8 g

- Protein: 3.3 g

Braised White Beans and Chard

Ingredients:

- ¼ bunch Swiss chard

- 1 Tbsp. olive oil

- ¼ medium yellow onion, diced

- 1 garlic clove, minced

- Salt and pepper

- ½ (15 oz.) can cannellini beans, drained and rinsed

- ½ cup vegetable broth

- 1 Tbsp. coarsely chopped fresh parsley

- 1 tsp. white wine vinegar

Directions:

1. Trim the ends from the chard stems and discard. Cut off the stems at the base of the

leaves and slice crosswise into 1/4-inch pieces; set aside. Stack the leaves and cut them into bite-size pieces; set aside.

2. Heat the oil in a Dutch oven or a heavy-bottomed pot over medium heat until shimmering. Add the chard stems, onion, and garlic and season with salt and pepper. Cook, stirring occasionally, until the vegetables have softened, about 8 minutes.

3. Add the chard leaves, beans, broth, and pinch of salt. Cook, stirring occasionally, until the leaves are wilted and the mixture has come to a simmer. Continue to simmer, stirring occasionally, until the chard is tender and the broth has thickened slightly, about 5 minutes more.

4. Remove from the heat and stir in the parsley and vinegar. Taste and season with salt and pepper as needed.

Nutritional Information

- Calories: 185

- Total Fat: 9 g

- Saturated Fat: 1.9 g

- Carbohydrates: 21 g

- Protein: 5 g

Miso Soup with Napa Cabbage

Ingredients:

- 1 tsp. olive oil

- ¼ medium yellow onion, thinly sliced

- 1 tsp. peeled, and finely chopped fresh ginger

- 1 garlic clove, minced

- 1 ½ cups vegetable broth

- ½ Tbsp. soy sauce

- ½ (12 oz.) package Udon Noodles

- ¼ medium napa cabbage, cored, halved lengthwise and cut into 1 inch pieces

- ½ carrot, julienned

- ¼ cup white miso

- Sriracha, or other chili sauce, for serving

Directions:

1. Bring a medium pot of heavily salted water to a boil over medium-high heat.

2. Add the udon to the pot of boiling water and cook according to the package directions. Drain in a colander and, while stirring, rinse the noodles with cold water until they're cooled and no longer sticky. Put the noodles in a deep bowl.

3. Meanwhile, heat the oil in a medium saucepan over medium heat until shimmering. Add the onion, ginger, garlic, and carrot, and cook, stirring occasionally, until the onions have softened, about 5 minutes.

4. Increase the heat to medium high. Add the broth and soy sauce and stir to combine.

5. Add the cabbage to the pan, stir to combine, and simmer until the cabbage is tender, about 5 minutes. Add the miso and stir to combine. Taste and season with salt as needed.

6. Top udon noodles with cabbage mixture and hot sauce, if desired.

Nutritional Information

- Calories: 130.9

- Total Fat: 2.1 g

- Saturated Fat: 0g

- Carbohydrates: 24g

- Protein: 4 g

Vegan Chinese Porridge

Ingredients:

- 2 cups water

- ½ cup vegetable broth

- ¼ cup long-grain brown rice

- ¼ inch piece of fresh ginger, skin on and sliced into 2 pieces

- Salt and white pepper

- 1 cup gai lan (known as Chinese broccoli or Chinese kale) ends trimmed and very thinly sliced (if you cannot find this, feel free to substitute regular broccoli

Directions:

1. Place all ingredients except the gai lan in a medium heavy-bottomed saucepan or Dutch oven and bring to a boil over medium-high heat. Reduce the heat to medium low and cook,

uncovered, at a lively simmer, stirring occasionally, until the rice has completely broken down and the mixture is creamy, about 1 1/2 hours.

2. Turn off the heat, add the gai lan, and stir until combined and the leaves are wilted.

3. Let sit until the residual heat cooks the gai lan stems to crisp-tender, about 5 minutes. Taste and season with additional salt and white pepper as needed.

Nutritional Information

- Calories: 146.1

- Total Fat: 0.9 g

- Saturated Fat: 0 g

- Carbohydrates: 31 g

- Protein: 3.5 g

Curried Carrot Soup

Ingredients:

- 1 tsp. olive oil

- 1 tsp. curry powder

- 1 garlic clove, smashed

- ¼ inch piece of ginger, peeled and smashed

- ¼ medium onion, coarsely chopped

- 2 carrots, peeled and sliced into ¼ inch thick rounds

- 1 bay leaf

- 1 cup vegetable broth

- ¼ cup canned coconut milk

Directions:

1. Heat the oil in a medium saucepan over medium heat. When it shimmers, add the curry powder and garlic and cook until fragrant, about 30 seconds.

2. Add the ginger, onion, carrots, bay leaf, and broth, increase the heat to medium high, and bring the mixture to a boil. Reduce the heat to medium low and simmer until the carrots are soft when pierced with a fork, about 20 minutes. Discard the bay leaf.

3. Working in batches, process the soup in a blender until smooth. (Be careful when blending the hot soup, as steam could blow off the blender lid.)

4. Pour the soup into a clean pot and return it to the stove over medium heat. Stir in the coconut milk and adjust the seasoning as needed. Serve hot.

Nutritional Information

- Calories: 249.8

- Total Fat: 13 g

- Saturated Fat: 11 g

- Carbohydrates: 30 g

- Protein: 3.2 g

Vegan Kofte

Ingredients:

- ¼ tsp ground coriander

- ¼ tsp ground cumin

- ¼-inch piece fresh ginger, peeled and chopped

- 1 clove garlic, minced

- ¼ zucchini, coarsely grated

- 1 tsp. olive oil

- Salt and pepper

- ¼ (15 oz.) can garbanzo beans

- 2 Tbsp. breadcrumbs

- 1 whole wheat pita

Minty-Yogurt Dip:

- 1/8 cucumber, roughly diced

- 1 sprig fresh mint, leaves removed and thinly sliced

- 1 Tbsp. soy yogurt (or other vegan yogurt)

- 1/4 lemon

Nutty Sauce:

- **Splash olive oil**

- **¼ small onion, diced**

- **1 clove garlic, diced**

- **¼ cup cashews**

- **2 Tbsp. light coconut milk**

- **½ Tbsp. smooth peanut butter**

Directions:

1. Heat oil in medium skillet over medium heat. Add ginger and garlic; fry 2-3 minutes, or until golden. Place in food processor, add cumin and coriander.

2. Place grated zucchini into a colander in the sink and sprinkle with salt. Squeeze the mixture together to get rid of excess moisture, then add to the processor.

3. Add garbanzo beans, breadcrumbs and a pinch of salt and pepper to the processor, pulse until combined, but not totally smooth.

4. Transfer to a clean work surface and with wet hands, divide and shape the mixture into 2-3 fat fingers. Place onto a plate and put in the fridge to chill for 20 minutes.

5. Meanwhile, make the minty-yogurt dip—place cucumber, yogurt, mint, and a squeeze of lemon juice in a bowl, mix well.

6. To make the nutty sauce—heat olive oil in a medium skillet over medium heat, add onion and garlic. Fry for 2-3 minutes. Add cashew and toast for 2-3 minutes. Transfer skillet contents to a food processor, add coconut milk and peanut butter and pulse until smooth.

7. Heat a splash of olive oil in a medium skillet over medium heat. Once hot, add kofte fingers from the fridge and cook for around 2 minutes, turning regularly. Serve with whole wheat pita and top with the two sauces.

Nutritional Information

- Calories: 270.7

- Total Fat: 11.1 g

- Saturated Fat: 2.8g

- Carbohydrates: 34.7g

- Protein: 8 g

Creamy Vegan Alfredo

Ingredients:

- ½ avocado, pitted
- Juice and zest from ¼ lemon
- 1 garlic clove, minced
- Pinch of salt and pepper
- 1 Tbsp. fresh basil, chopped
- 1 Tbsp. fresh parsley, chopped
- 1 Tbsp. extra virgin olive oil
- 2 ½ Tbsp. walnuts, chopped and toasted, for garnish
- Fresh parsley, for garnish
- ½ cup dry pasta (any kind)

Directions:

1. Start by bringing a small pot of salted water to a boil. Add your pasta of choice and cover, cooking 7-10 minutes until done. Drain and set aside.

2. Meanwhile, make the sauce by placing lemon juice, garlic, and olive oil in a food processor. Blend until fairly smooth.

3. Add basil, parsley, avocado, salt and pepper. Process until very smooth.

4. Toss the pasta with the sauce and garnish with fresh parsley, lemon zest, and walnuts.

Nutritional Information

- Calories: 388

- Total Fat: 20 g

- Saturated Fat: 3 g

- Carbohydrates:42 g

- Protein: 10 g

We appreciate you ordering our books. We try and provide only the best natural solutions that we have found proof that they can be of benefit. If you would be so kind as to please leave a review for our book we would appreciate it greatly. The only way to help others is to spread the message yourself once you find something that helps.

We can understand if some of the recipes inside of this book may not be for you, or they may not do much in relieving your specific gout problem.

We are truly sorry for that and hope that you can ultimately find your solution for your specific gout problem.

We do hope that you will also understand that many people are finding gout relief through utilizing our recipes. We have helped thousands of people relieve their gout flair ups all through a proper diet.

Remember, when you find what works for you the main thing is to be consistent with it. This is the only way for you to hopefully one day rid yourself of the worst this painful disease can often bring.

Thank you.

Disclaimer:

The information provided in this book is designed to provide helpful information on the subjects discussed. This book is not meant to be used, nor should it be used, to diagnose or treat any medical condition. For diagnosis or treatment of any medical problem, consult your own physician. The publisher and author are not responsible for any specific health or allergy needs that may require medical supervision and are not liable for any damages or negative consequences from any treatment, action, application or preparation, to any person reading or following the information in this book. References are provided for informational purposes only and do not constitute endorsement of any websites or other sources. Readers should be aware that the websites listed in this book may change.

Check out this title exclusively on Amazon by HR Research Alliance that can give real answers to that age old mystery known as ERECTILE DYSFUNCTION.

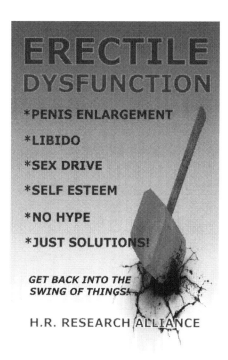

Finally a natural remedy that actually works!

21287450R00097

Made in the USA
Middletown, DE
24 June 2015